Copyright 2023

All right reserved. No part of this book should be resproduce without express permission of the author.

Reproduction of all or any part of this book is punishable under relevant law.

Table of Contents

PREVIEW

Eczema is a condition in which patches of skin become inflamed, itchy, cracked, and rough. Some types can also cause blisters. Home remedies and medical treatment can help manage and prevent flares.

Different types and stages of <u>eczema</u> affect <u>31.6 million</u> people in the United States, which equals more than 10% of the population.

Many people use the word eczema when referring to atopic dermatitis, which is the most common type. The term atopic refers to a collection of conditions that involve the immune system, including atopic dermatitis, asthma, and <u>hay fever</u>. The word dermatitis refers to inflammation of the skin.

Certain foods, such as nuts and dairy, can trigger symptoms of eczema. Environmental triggers can include smoke, pollen, soaps, and fragrances. Eczema is not contagious.

About a <u>quarter</u> of children in the U.S. have the condition, as well as <u>10%</u> of African Americans, 13% of Asian Americans and Pacific Islanders, 13% of Native Americans, and 11% of people who are white.

Some people outgrow the condition, while others will continue to have it throughout adulthood. This article will explain what eczema is and discuss its symptoms, treatments, causes, and types.

ECZEMA DIET RECIPES

BREAKFAST

1. Pear Pea Protein Muffins

Prep Time: 10 Minutes

Cook Time: 20 Minutes

Serving: 12

Ingredients

- 1 tbsp flax seeds
- 1 1/4 cups spelt flour
- 3/4 cup 100% pure pea protein powder
- 3 tsp baking powder
- 1/2 tsp baking soda
- pinch fine sea salt
- 1/2 cup barley malt syrup (my favorite!) or rice syrup
- 1 cup filtered water
- 1/2 tsp pure vanilla extract or 1/8 tsp ground vanilla bean (optional)
- 1/3 cup virgin sunflower oil or rice bran oil
- 2 pears, peeled and diced

Instructions

1. Grind flax seeds and mix with 3tbsp water. Set aside until gelatinous.
2. In a large bowl, mix spelt flour, pea protein powder, baking powder, baking soda and sea salt.
3. In a blender, add syrup, water, vanilla and flax seed mixture. Blend until combined. Keep blender on low speed and slowly add in oil.
4. Add liquid ingredients to dry ingredients and mix until combined.
5. Mix in peeled diced pear.
6. Fill muffin cups and bake for 18-20 minutes, or until a toothpick inserted in the centre comes out clean.
7. Let cool for 5 minutes in the pan, then transfer to a cooling rack.

2. Cranberry, Apple & Rosemary Breakfast Cakes

Prep Time: 10 Minutes

Cook Time: 20 Minutes

Serving: 12

Ingredients

- 1 1/2 cups whole wheat pastry flour
- 1/2 cup almond flour
- 1/4 cup cane sugar
- 1 tbsp baking powder
- 1/2 tsp fine sea salt
- 2 big sprigs of rosemary, stem removed and very finely chopped
- 1/2 cup applesauce
- 3/4 cup unsweetened almond milk
- 1 cup fresh cranberries
- 1 medium apple, chopped (yields approximately 1 cup; I used McIntosh)

Instructions

1. In a large bowl, combine whole wheat pastry flour, almond flour, sugar, baking powder, salt and rosemary.
2. Add applesauce and mix until incorporated and flour mixture is crumbly (you might have to use your hands).
3. Add the almond milk and stir with a spoon until incorporated and you have a homogenous batter, without over mixing.
4. Stir in cranberries and chopped apple.
5. Use a 1/4 cup measure to drop batter on your baking sheet. Leave some space (I would say at least 2 inches) between each cake as they double in size while baking.
6. Bake for 20 minutes, or until lightly golden. Transfer to a cooling rack.

3. Coconut, Applesauce & Dark Chocolate Chunk Oat Bars

Prep Time: 40 Minutes

Cook Time: 10 Minutes

Serving: 8

Ingredients

- 1/4 cup milk (I used unsweetened almond milk)
- 1/2 cup unpacked brown sugar
- 1 tbsp flax seeds, grounded
- 1 tbsp chia seeds
- 1/4 cup coconut oil, melted
- 1 tsp pure vanilla extract
- 1/2 cup unsweetened applesauce
- 1 1/2 cups rolled oats
- 1/2 cup unsweetened shredded coconut
- 1/2 tsp grounded cinnamon
- 1/4 cup whole wheat flour
- 1/2 tsp baking powder
- 1/8 tsp fine sea salt
- 1/3 cup chopped dark chocolate (I used 85%)

Instruction

1. In a bowl, whisk almond milk, sugar, grounded flax, chia seeds, melted coconut oil, vanilla and applesauce together and set aside. In a second bowl, mix oats, coconut, cinnamon, flour, baking powder and salt. Add to the wet mixture and stir with a wooden spoon until combined. Stir in chopped chocolate.

2. Scoop half the batter in each bread pan. Smooth out and press down firmly with a spatula. Bake for 35-40 minutes, until the edges begin to get golden. Cool 10 minutes in the pans, then transfer to a wire rack (remove using the parchment paper hanging on the sides) to cool completely. Slice each half in four bars.

4. Carrot Wheat Bran Muffins

Prep Time: 10 Minutes

Cook Time: 20 Minutes

Serving: 9

Ingredients

- 1 tbsp cider vinegar + almond milk to make 1 cup
- 1 1/2 cups wheat bran
- 1 flax egg (1 tbsp flax seeds, grounded + 3 tbsp water)
- 1/3 cup applesauce
- 1/3 cup brown sugar
- 1/2 tsp vanilla extract
- 1 cup whole wheat flour
- 1 tsp baking soda
- 1 tsp baking powder
- 1/2 tsp fine sea salt
- 1 tsp ground cinnamon
- 1 1/2 cups grated carrots
- 1/3 cup raisins
- 1/4 cup pecans, chopped

Instructions

1. In a measuring cup, add 1 tbsp apple cider
   vinegar, then fill with almond milk to make 1
   cup. Stir and set aside a couple minutes until
   curdled. Then, add almond milk mixture to
   wheat bran, stir well and wet aside for 10
   minutes.
2. Meanwhile, prepare flax egg by whisking
   grounded flax and water. Set aside.
3. Preheat oven to 375°F. Line a muffin tin with
   paper liners. When the wheat bran mixture is
   ready, beat flax egg, applesauce, sugar and
   vanilla with a hand mixer. Beat in wheat bran
   mixture. In an other bowl, mix flour, baking
   soda, baking powder, salt and cinnamon. Add
   the dry ingredients to the wet ingredients and
   stir with a wooden spoon until combined. Stir in
   grated carrots, raisins and pecans.
4. Spoon the batter in the prepared muffin tins.
   Bake for 20 minutes, or until a toothpick
   inserted in the center comes out clean. Let cool
   5 minutes in the muffin tin before transferring
   to a cooling rack.

5. Juicy Blueberry Muffins

Prep Time: 5 Minutes

Cook Time: 15 Minutes

Serving: 12

Ingredients

- 1 cup whole wheat pastry flour
- 1/2 cup unbleached all purpose flour
- 1/4 cup packed brown sugar
- 1/4 cup organic cane sugar
- 1/4 cup wheat germ
- 1/4 cup rolled oats
- 1/2 tsp ground cinnamon
- 1/4 tsp ground nutmeg
- 1/8 tsp ground cardamom
- 1 tsp baking powder
- 1 tsp baking soda
- 1/4 tsp fine sea salt
- 1 cup fresh blueberries
- 3/4 cup unsweetened applesauce
- 1/2 cup buttermilk
- 1/2 cup plain Greek yogurt

- 1 tbsp safflower oil (or canola/vegetable)
- 1 tsp pure vanilla extract

Instructions

1. In a large bowl, stir flours, sugars, wheat germ, oats, spices, baking powder, baking soda and salt. Gently stir in the blueberries.
2. In a second bowl, whisk applesauce, buttermilk, yogurt, oil and vanilla. Add to dry ingredients and stir until just combined. Spoon into muffin cups, filing all the way to the top. Bake for 20-22 minutes, or until the tops of the muffins spring back when lightly touched.

6. Peanut Butter, Banana & Dark Chocolate Muffins

Prep Time: 5 Minutes

Cook Time: 18 Minutes

Serving: 12

Ingredients

- 1 cup spelt flour
- 1/2 cup whole wheat flour
- 1/4 cup organic cane sugar
- 2 tsp baking powder
- 1/2 tsp fine sea salt
- 1/2 cup all-natural smooth peanut butter
- 1/4 cup earth balance, or other non-hydrogenated margarine
- 3/4 cup milk (I used unsweetened vanilla almond milk)
- 1 large ripe banana, mashed
- 6 tsp dark chocolate peanut butter

Instructions

1. In a large bowl, mix flours, sugar, baking powder and salt with a whisk. Add peanut butter and earth balance

and mix with hands until it looks like crumble. Add milk and mashed banana and stir with a wooden spoon until combined. Spoon the batter in the prepared muffin cups.

2. Add 1/2 tsp of dark chocolate peanut butter in the middle of each muffin and swirl with a toothpick. Bake for 15-18 minutes, or until a toothpick comes out clean. Cool in pan for 5 minutes before transferring to wire rack.

7. Lemon Poppy Seed Bread with Pomegranate Glaze

Prep Time: 60 Minutes

Cook Time: 10 Minutes

Serving: 1

Ingredients

- 1/2 cup earth balance (or butter), softened
- 3/4 cup golden cane sugar
- 1 tbsp agave nectar
- 2 flax eggs, divided
- 1/2 cup milk (I used unsweetened almond milk)
- Zest of 1 lemon
- 1/2 tsp lemon extract
- 1/2 tsp fine sea salt
- 3/4 cup unbleached all purpose flour
- 3/4 cup whole wheat flour
- 1 tsp baking powder
- 3 tbsp poppy seeds

Glaze:

- 1/4 cup POM wonderful pomegranate juice
- 1/4 cup golden cane sugar

- 1 tbsp agave nectar

Instructions

1. Prepare flax eggs: in a small bowl, mix 1 tbsp flax seeds, grounded, and 3 tbsp water. Repeat to have two divided flax eggs and set aside.
2. In a bowl, combine flours, salt and baking powder with a whisk.
3. Beat earth balance with a hand mixer until fluffy, about 1-2 minutes. Add sugar and agave, continue to beat until creamy. Add flax eggs, one at a time, beating after each addition to incorporate. On low speed, slowly beat in the milk, then mix in lemon zest and extract. Slowly add in dry ingredients and beat until smooth. Place the batter in the prepared pan and bake for 1 hour.
4. While the bread is baking, prepare the glaze: place all the glaze ingredients in a small saucepan and heat on low until sugar is completely dissolved.
5. When you remove the bread from the oven, poke holes all over the top with a toothpick. Spoon the glaze over the bread while it is still hot and in the pan. Let cool for 10 minutes before removing from the pan.

8. Raspberry Whole Grain Scones with Cream Cheese Frosting Cream And Jam

Prep Time: 5 Minutes

Cook Time: 22 Minutes

Serving: 8

Ingredients

- 1 cup spelt flour
- 1 cup rolled oats
- 1/4 cup unpacked brown sugar
- 1/4 tsp fine sea salt
- 2 tsp baking powder
- 1/2 tsp baking soda
- 1/4 cup safflower oil (or canola)
- 1/4 cup vanilla yogurt (I used 2.5% M.F.)
- 3 tbsp milk (I used almond milk)
- 1 tsp vanilla extract
- 1/3 cup frozen raspberries
- Turbinado sugar, to garnish
- Berry jam of your choice (I used strawberry)

Frosting cream:

- 2 tbsp earth balance (or butter), at room temperature
- 1/4 cup cream cheese
- 3 tbsp icing sugar

Instructions

1. In a food processor grind the oats until a flour consistency is achieved. In a large bowl, whisk together the spelt flour, oat flour, sugar, salt, baking powder, and baking soda. Add in the oil and mix with hands until it looks like crumble.
2. In a second bowl, whisk together the yogurt, milk and vanilla. Add to the dry mixture and stir until just combined. Add frozen raspberries and mix until just combined.
3. Spoon 1/4 cup batter per scone onto the prepared baking sheet. Sprinkle with turbinado sugar and bake for 20-22 minutes, until golden.
4. While the scones are baking, make your frosting by whisking (by hand) all ingredients together. At first, it will look like it won't work but it will transform into a yummy frosting quickly.

5. After scones are done, let cool 5 minutes on baking
   sheets and serve with a big spoon of frosting and a little
   ja

9. Maple Espresso Scones

Prep Time: 60 Minutes

Cook Time: 18 Minutes

Serving: 8

Ingredients

- 3 1/4 cups unbleached all purpose flour
- 2/3 cup golden cane sugar
- 5 tsp baking powder
- 1/4 tsp fine sea salt
- 3/4 cup earth balance (or softened butter)
- 1 flax egg: mix 1 tbsp flax seeds, grounded, and 3 tbsp water
- 1 tbsp maple extract/flavoring
- 3/4 cup milk (I used unsweetened almond milk)
- 1 tbsp instant espresso mixed with 1/2 tsp water

Glaze:

- 1/2 cup icing sugar
- 1/8 cup maple syrup
- 3/4 tsp maple extract/flavoring

Instructions

1. Prepare flax egg and instant espresso mixture and set aside.

2. In a bowl, combine flour, sugar, baking powder and salt. Add earth balance and mix with your hands until crumbly. In a second bowl, whisk flax egg, maple extract, milk and espresso mixture. Add to dry ingredients and combine with your hands.

3. Make a ball with the dough and transfer to a floured surface. Knead the dough 10 times with floured hands. Pat the dough into a 8-inch circle. Cut the dough to make 8 triangular scones. Transfer scones to baking sheet and bake for 18 minutes. Let cool.

4. When the scones are cooled, combine all the glaze ingredients with a whisk until combined. Spread on the scones with a knife and let set for an hour.

10. Granola Pumpkin Bars

Prep Time: 30 Minutes

Cook Time: 5 Minutes

Serving: 8

Ingredients

- 3 cups rolled oats
- 1 cup walnut pieces
- ¼ cup pumpkin seeds
- 1 tsp. pumpkin pie spices
- Pinch of salt
- ½ cup canned pumpkin
- ½ cup applesauce
- ½ cup maple syrup

Instructions

1. In a medium bowl measure 3 cups oats. Add 1 cup walnut pieces, ¼ cup pumpkin seeds, 1 tsp. pumpkin pie spices and a pinch of salt. Mix them all.

2. Now measure the wet ingredients. ½ cup canned pumpkin, ½ cup applesauce and ½ cup maple syrup.

Add them to the dry ingredients and mix until combined.

3. Spread mixture evenly into the baking pan. Bake in preheated oven approximately 30 minutes until golden brown. Let cool for 5 minutes and cut into bars using a sharp knife.

LUNCH

11. Roasted Brussels Sprouts Pasta with Mung Bean Sprouts

Prep Time: 10 Minutes

Cook Time: 40 Minutes

Serving: 4

Ingredients

- 4 heaping cups Brussels sprouts, quartered
- 1 leek, halved lengthwise and sliced
- 2 cloves garlic, pressed
- 2 tbsp virgin sunflower oil or rice bran oil, divided
- 1lb package of spelt, rice or quinoa pasta (I used whole spelt fusilli)
- salt to taste
- 1/4 cup mung bean sprouts

Instructions

1. Add Brussels sprouts, leek and garlic to an oven-safe casserole dish. Add 1 tbsp of oil and salt to taste and mix. Cover with a lid or aluminum foil, making sure

there is still space in the dish (or the Brussels sprouts won't cook as well).

2. Bake in the preheated oven for 40 minutes.
3. Meanwhile, fill a big pot of water with water and bring to a boil.
4. When there is approximately 10 minutes left for the Brussels sprouts to bake, cook pasta according to package directions.
5. Drain pasta and add back to pot.
6. Add remaining 1 tbsp of oil, baked vegetables and salt to taste, and toss to mix well.
7. Serve topped with mung bean sprouts.

12. Red Lentil Cabbage Soup

Prep Time: 15 Minutes

Cook Time: 40 Minutes

Serving: 6

Ingredients

- 1 leek, finely diced
- 3 cloves garlic, minced or pressed
- 1 large (or 1 1/2 small) green cabbage, coarsely chopped
- 3 cups chopped green beans
- 1 1/2 cups red lentils, rinsed
- 4 tbsp spelt flour (use buckwheat or brown rice flour for a gluten-free soup)
- salt to taste

Instructions

1. Add leek and garlic to a big pot with a couple tablespoons of water. Sautée on medium heat until soft.

2. Add cabbage and green beans. Add water and/or vegetable broth until you cover the vegetables by 1-inch.

3. Bring to a boil. Lower heat, cover, and simmer for 15-20 minutes.

4. Add red lentils, mix, bring back to a boil, lower heat and simmer uncovered for 15 more minutes.

5. Whisk flour with about 1/4 cup of water. Add to the soup and mix well. Let simmer a couple more minutes and remove from heat. Add salt to taste.

6. The soup is even better the next day!

13. Oat Groats, Lentil & Roasted Brussels Sprouts Salad

Prep Time: 20 Minutes

Cook Time: 45 Minutes

Serving: 6

Ingredients

- 1 1/2 cups oat groats (see note)
- 1 cup brown lentils
- 650g Brussels Sprouts, quartered
- 1 leek, sliced lengthwise, then chopped in 1/4 inch slices
- 1 1/2 tbsp virgin sunflower oil or rice bran oil
- 1/4 tsp garlic powder (no additives)
- 2 green onions, green parts only, finely sliced
- 3 tsp flax oil
- salt to taste

Instructions

1. Add oat groats to a pot full of water. Bring to a boil, reduce heat, cover and cook for 45-50 minutes. Drain.

2. Add lentils to a pot with 3 cups of water. Bring to a boil, reduce heat, cover and cook for 30 minutes. Remove from heat and keep covered until oat groats are ready. If there is some water left, drain.

3. Add Brussels sprouts, leeks, sunflower or rice bran oil, garlic powder and a couple pinches of salt to a big oven-safe casserole dish. Mix well. Cover with a lid or aluminum paper and bake at 425°F for 35-40 minutes.

4. When oat groats, lentils and Brussels sprouts are ready, transfer to a bowl. Let cool until room temperature (or close). Add green onions, flax oil and salt to taste and mix.

14. Lemony Quinoa Salad with Zucchini Ribbons

Prep Time: 5 Minutes

Cook Time: 12 Minutes

Serving: 2

Ingredients

- 1/2 cup quinoa
- 1 cipollini onion, chopped
- 1/2 tsp sriracha sauce
- 1 zucchini
- Sea salt
- 1/2 cup chopped red cabbage
- 1 cup chopped tomato
- 1/2 cup chopped sweet pepper
- 1/4 cup crumbled feta cheese
- 1/4 cup raisins
- Juice of 1 lemon
- 1 tbsp extra virgin olive oil
- 1/2 tbsp raw honey

Instructions

1. Rinse quinoa. Add to a saucepan with 3/4 cup water, the chopped onion and sriracha and bring to a boil. Redude heat to low, cover and let cook 12 minutes. Remove from heat and let stand 5 minutes. Transfer to a bowl to cool.

2. Meanwhile, cut both ends of the zucchini. Using a vegetable peeler, slice zucchini lengthwise to make the ribbons. You can also use a mandoline if you have one. Put zucchini in a strainer and sprinkle with fine sea salt. Toss with hands and let zucchini drain for 15 minutes, then pat dry.

3. When the quinoa is cooled, mix it with the red cabbage, tomato, sweet pepper, feta and raisins. In a small bowl, whisk lemon juice, olive oil and honey together. Add to the quinoa and toss until well coated. Add the zucchini ribbons and toss gently.

15. Easy 4-Bean Salad

Prep Time: 00 Minutes

Cook Time: 00 Minutes

Serving: 7

Ingredients

- 1 can (14 oz) no salt added cut wax beans
- 1 can (14 oz) no salt added cut green beans
- 1 can (19 oz) chickpeas, drained and rinsed
- 1 can (19 oz) red kidney beans, drained and rinsed
- 1 orange bell pepper, chopped
- 1 celery stalk, very finely chopped
- 1/3 cup packed chopped flat-leaf parsley
- 3 green onions, chopped

Dressing:

- 4 tbsp lemon juice
- 2 tbsp lime juice
- 2 tbsp walnut oil, or oil of choice
- 1 tbsp red wine vinegar
- 1 tbsp pure maple syrup

- 1 tbsp old-style (grainy) mustard

- 1 tsp white balsamic vinegar

- 1/2 tsp yellow mustard

- 2 drops tabasco

- 1 tbsp hulled hemp seeds

- salt and pepper to taste

Instructions

1. In a large bowl, combine toss all salad ingredients together. In a small bowl, whisk all the dressing ingredients together. Pour on salad and mix well. Place in fridge until ready to serve (the salad is better the next day). Store in an air-tight container in the fridge for up to one week.

16. Quinoa Lime Biryani

Prep Time: 20 Minutes

Cook Time: 00 Minutes

Serving: 4

Ingredients

- 2 limes
- 1 cup dry quinoa
- 1 1/4 cup water
- 2 1/2 tbsp olive oil
- 1 tsp hot curry powder
- 1/8 tsp ground cinnamon
- 1/8 tsp ground ginger
- 3/4 tsp fine sea salt
- 1/4 cup sliced almonds
- 1 can (15 oz) chickpeas, rinsed and drained
- 1/2 bunch scallions, thinly sliced
- 1 large (or 2 small-medium) carrot, grated on the medium grating surface
- 1/4 cup dried currants
- Black pepper to taste

Instructions

2. Juice one lime. In a saucepan, combine the lime juice, quinoa, water, 1/2 tbsp olive oil, spices and 1/2 tsp salt. Bring to a boil, reduce heat, stir, cover and simmer for 15 to 20 minutes, until all the liquid is absorbed. Transfer to a large bowl and let cool.
3. In a skillet over medium heat, toast the sliced almonds until golden.
4. When the quinoa is at room temperature, toss in carrots, chickpeas, scallions, almonds and currants.
5. Zest and juice the second lime. In a small bowl, combine the zest and juice with the remaining 2 tbsp oil, 1/4 tsp salt and pepper to taste. Pour on the quinoa and toss.
6. You can make the salad 1-2 day(s) in advance.

17. Quick & Easy Pasta Carbonara

Prep Time: 00 Minutes

Cook Time: 00 Minutes

Serving: 4

Ingredients

- 4 servings (375g) whole wheat linguine (or other pasta of your choice)
- 8 slices vegetarian bacon
- 1 cup 15% thick country cream
- 2 egg yolks
- 1/2 tsp dried parsley flakes
- Grated parmesan, to taste
- Freshly ground black pepper, to tast

Instructions

1. Bring a pot of water to a boil. Add pasta and cook according to package directions.
2. Meanwhile, cook bacon according to package directions. Break it in small pieces. In a big bowl, whisk egg yolks and cream together.

3. When pasta is ready, drain and transfer to the bowl. Toss to coat with the sauce. Add bacon and toss again. Serve immediately sprinkled with parmesan and black pepper.

18. Colorful Bean Sprout Salad

Prep Time: 3hrs 00 Minutes

Cook Time: 00 Minutes

Serving: 4

Ingredients

- 500 g (60 oz) bean sprouts
- 2 celery stalks, chopped
- 2 carrots, peeled and chopped
- 1 bell pepper, seeds removed, chopped
- 1 tomato, diced
- 15 green beans, ends removed, coarsely chopped

Vinaigrette:

- 1/2 cup low sodium soy sauce (or tamari/coconut aminos)
- 2 tbsp olive oil
- juice of 1/2 lemon
- 1/4 cup honey (maple syrup might work for vegans)
- 1 clove garlic, pressed

Instructions

1. Prepare all veggies and put them in a big salad bowl. In a small bowl, whisk the vinaigrette ingredients together. Pour on the veggies and toss. Cover with plastic wrap and marinate for at least 3 hours (I always make it the day before), tossing a couple of times.

19. Ratatouille

Prep Time: 1hrs 30 Minutes

Cook Time: 10 Minutes

Serving: 5

Ingredients

- 5 tbsp olive oil
- 2 big spanish onions, coarsely chopped
- 3 bell peppers, coarsely chopped
- 1 eggplant, cut in half and sliced
- 4 green zucchinis, sliced
- 2 yellow zucchinis, sliced
- 2 cans (28 ounces) crushed tomatoes
- 5 cloves garlic, pressed
- 2 bay leafs
- Salt, pepper to taste

Instructions

1. In a large pot (at least 6-quart), heat oil over medium heat. Add onion and cook, stirring frequently, until it begins to get translucent. Add bell peppers and cook for

5 more minutes. Add zucchinis and eggplant and cook
for 5 more minutes. Add tomatoes, bay leafs, garlic, salt
and pepper and stir. Reduce heat to low, cover and let
simmer 1 hour, then 30 minutes uncovered.

20. Casserole and Cookies

Prep Time: 00 Minutes

Cook Time: 15 Minutes

Serving: 10

Ingredients

- 1 cup spelt flour
- 1 tsp baking powder
- 1/2 tsp baking soda
- 1/4 cup unrefined cane sugar
- 1/8 tsp fine sea salt
- 1/3 cup maple syrup
- 1/2 tbsp maple extract
- 1/3 cup safflower oil
- 1/3 cup chopped walnuts

Instructions

1. In a bowl, mix dry ingredients (flour, baking powder, baking soda, sugar and salt). In a second bowl, whisk together maple syrup and maple extract. Add oil and

whisk until homogeneous. Add dry ingredients and mix until fully incorporated. Mix in walnuts.

2. Line 1-2 baking sheet(s) with parchment paper. Make 1 tbsp balls of dough and place on baking sheet (leave as much space as possible between them). Bake for 15 minutes, or until golden brown.

DINNER

21. Quinoa Lime Biryani

Prep Time: 20 Minutes

Cook Time: 00 Minutes

Serving: 4

Ingredients

- 2 limes
- 1 cup dry quinoa
- 1 1/4 cup water
- 2 1/2 tbsp olive oil
- 1 tsp hot curry powder
- 1/8 tsp ground cinnamon
- 1/8 tsp ground ginger
- 3/4 tsp fine sea salt
- 1/4 cup sliced almonds
- 1 can (15 oz) chickpeas, rinsed and drained
- 1/2 bunch scallions, thinly sliced
- 1 large (or 2 small-medium) carrot, grated on the medium grating surface
- 1/4 cup dried currants
- Black pepper to taste

Instructions

1. Juice one lime. In a saucepan, combine the lime juice, quinoa, water, 1/2 tbsp olive oil, spices and 1/2 tsp salt. Bring to a boil, reduce heat, stir, cover and simmer for 15 to 20 minutes, until all the liquid is absorbed. Transfer to a large bowl and let cool.
2. In a skillet over medium heat, toast the sliced almonds until golden.
3. When the quinoa is at room temperature, toss in carrots, chickpeas, scallions, almonds and currants.
4. Zest and juice the second lime. In a small bowl, combine the zest and juice with the remaining 2 tbsp oil, 1/4 tsp salt and pepper to taste. Pour on the quinoa and toss.
5. You can make the salad 1-2 day(s) in advance

22. Baked Pumpkin Mac & Cheese

Prep Time: 5 Minutes

Cook Time: 30 Minutes

Serving: 4

Ingredients

- 1 tbsp olive oil
- 1 white onion, chopped
- 1 package (375 g) whole wheat elbow macaroni
- 2 slices of bread (I used sprouted whole wheat)
- 3 tbsp softened butter (or non-hydrogenated margarine), divided
- 1 tbsp flour (I used whole wheat)
- 1 cup warm milk (I used 1%)
- 1/2 package Maclaren's Imperial Sharp Cold Pack Cheddar
- 2/3 cup pumpkin puree
- 1/8 tsp ground nutmeg
- 1 tsp salted herbs, or salt to taste
- 1/2 cup shredded cheese of your choice (I used Oka Classique)
- Paprika

Instructions

1. Heat olive oil in a skillet over medium heat. Cook onion until it starts to brown. Remove from heat and set aside.

2. Bring a big pot of water to a boil and cook macaroni according to package instructions.

3. Meanwhile, process the two slices of bread in a food processor until coarse crumbs start to form. Add 2 tbsp softened butter and process until combined. Set aside.

4. In a large saucepan, melt remaining 1 tbsp butter over medium heat. Add flour and stir with a whisk until it starts to bubble. Whisk in milk, then stir constantly until sauce begins to thicken, about 5 minutes.

5. Add cheese and stir until completely melted. Add pumpkin, nutmeg and salted herbs. Toss the drained macaroni and cooked onions in the sauce.

6. Transfer macaroni 4 individual baking dishes. Top with shredded cheese, then with bread crumbs and sprinkle with paprika. Bake for 30 minutes and serve immediatel

23. Creamy Mushroom Gnocchi

Prep Time: 3 Minutes

Cook Time: 4 Minutes

Serving: 4

Ingredients

- 2 tbsp olive oil
- 1 tbsp butter
- 2 cups sliced cremini mushrooms
- 3 cloves garlic, pressed
- 1/2 tsp dried parsley
- 1/2 tsp dried thyme
- 1 cup vegetable broth
- 1/4 cup cream
- 1 tbsp cornstarch mixed with 1 tbsp water
- 1 package (500g) gnocchi
- Parmesan cheese (optional)

Instructions

1. Bring a large pot of water to a boil. Meanwhile, make
   your sauce.

2. Melt butter with olive oil in a saucepan over medium heat. Add mushrooms, garlic, parsley and thyme and cook until tender. Add stock an increase to medium-high heat. Once the stock comes to a boil, reduce to medium heat and add cream and cornstarch mixture. Bring back to a boil and cook on medium-low for 2-4 minutes.

3. Add gnocchi to boiling water and cook according to package directions (usually takes 2-3 minutes, like the sauce!

4. Add gnocchi to the sauce and mix. Serve garnished with parmesan if desired.

24. Vegan Stuffed Peppers

Prep Time: 25 Minutes

Cook Time: 3 Minutes

Serving: 3

Ingredients

- 1/3 cup dry quinoa (I mixed red and white)
- 3 small to medium bell peppers
- 1-2 tbsp olive oil
- 2 carrots, diced
- 1/4 white onion, chopped
- 1 clove garlic
- 1 cup frozen spinach (5 nuggets), thawed and drained
- 1 cup canned or cooked red kidney beans
- 1/2 tsp chili powder

Instructions

1. Cook quinoa according to package directions.
2. Preheat oven to 375°F. Heat oil in a skillet over medium-low heat. Add carrots, cook for 3 minutes. Add onion and garlic and cook until the onion is

translucent. Remove from heat, add beans and spinach and toss well. Add quinoa and chili powder.

3. Cut the top off the peppers and remove the seeds. Fill them with the quinoa mixture and replace tops. Put in a baking dish, add just enough water to coat the bottom and bake for 20-25 minutes. Serve immediately.

25. Sweet Potato Green Bean Casserole

Prep Time: 20 Minutes

Cook Time: 1hr 5 Minutes

Serving: 5

Ingredients

- 3 tbsp vegan butter (such as Earth Balance)
- 1 tsp neutral tasting oil + more to brush the sweet potato
- 1 large vidalia onion or 2 sweet onions, thinly sliced
- 1 large sweet potato, peeled and sliced
- 1 pound green beans, ends trimmed
- Florets from 1 small or ½ large cauliflower
- 1 package (12.3oz) firm silken tofu, drained
- 1 cup non-dairy milk
- 1 ½ tbsp nutritional yeast
- 1 tsp salt + more to taste
- 2 tsp cornstarch

Pinch or freshly ground nutmeg

- 2 cloves garlic, pressed or minced
- 1 package (8oz) cremini mushrooms, finely diced
- 1 tsp dried thyme
- ¼ cup dry white wine
- 2 bread slices
- Black pepper to taste

Instructions

1. The caramelized onions:Melt 2 tbsp of vegan butter over medium-low heat. Add the sliced onion and let cook for about an hour until caramelized, while Make completing the other steps. Stir occasionally.
2. Prep the sweet potatoes:Spread the sweet potato slices on a baking sheet and brush both sides with oil. Lightly sprinkle with salt. Bake for 40 minutes, turning halfway through.
3. Prep the green beans:
4. Steam the green beans for 6-7 minutes and transfer to ice water.

5. Make the mushroom soup:

6. Steam the cauliflower for about 15 minutes, until very soft.

7. In a blender, add the steamed cauliflower, tofu, non-dairy milk, nutritional yeasttarch and pinch of nutmeg. Process until completely smooth.

8. In a large saucepan, heat 1 tbsp of vegan butter and 1 tsp of oil over medium heat.

9. Add garlic and sautée for 1-2 minutes. Add the diced mushrooms and sautée until soft and water has evaporated. Add thyme and sautée for 30 more seconds.

10. Add white wine and cook until evaporated. Add the cauliflower mixture and keep over medium heat. When the mixture is hot and starts to boil, reduce to low heat. Let cook for 15 minutes. Add salt and pepper to taste.

11. Make the casserole:In a 9×13 inch casserole dish, spread the roasted sweet potato slices. Top with the green beans. Pour the mushroom soup on top and spread to cover all the vegetables.Put the caramelized onions in paper towels and squeeze out the excess of vegan butter. Spread on top of the mushroom soup.Put the two bread

slices in a food processor and process to get bread crumbs. Sprinkle on top of the casserole.Bake for 20 minutes.

26. Pear Coleslaw

Prep Time: 15 Minutes

Cook Time: 00 Minutes

Serving: 6

Ingredients

- 4 cups thinly sliced red and green cabbage
- 3/4 tsp fine celtic salt or fine sea salt
- 3 green onions, green parts only, sliced
- 2 ripe pears, peeled
- 1/2 tbsp virgin sunflower oil (see note)

Instructions

1. Place the cabbage in a bowl. Add salt and massage the cabbage. Set aside to soften for 5 minutes. Add the green onions, massage again and set aside 5-10 minutes.
2. Thinly slice 1 1/2 pear. Add to the cabbage.
3. Mash the remaining 1/2 pear. Mix in the oil. Pour on the salad, mix and serve.

27. Red Lentil Cabbage Soup

Prep Time: 15 Minutes

Cook Time: 40 Minutes

Serving: 6

Ingredients

- 1 leek, finely diced
- 3 cloves garlic, minced or pressed
- 1 large (or 1 1/2 small) green cabbage, coarsely chopped
- 3 cups chopped green beans
- 1 1/2 cups red lentils, rinsed
- 4 tbsp spelt flour (use buckwheat or brown rice flour for a gluten-free soup)
- salt to taste

Instructions

1. Add leek and garlic to a big pot with a couple tablespoons of water. Sautée on medium heat until soft.

2. Add cabbage and green beans. Add water and/or vegetable broth until you cover the vegetables by 1-inch.

3. Bring to a boil. Lower heat, cover, and simmer for 15-20 minutes.

4. Add red lentils, mix, bring back to a boil, lower heat and simmer uncovered for 15 more minutes.

5. Whisk flour with about 1/4 cup of water. Add to the soup and mix well. Let simmer a couple more minutes and remove from heat. Add salt to taste.

6. The soup is even better the next day!

28. Double-Banana Chocolate Chip Oat Squares

Prep Time: 10 Minutes

Cook Time: 20 Minutes

Serving: 12

Ingredients

- 1 flax egg: mix 1 tbsp flax seeds, grounded, with 3 tbsp water and set aside
- 1 very ripe banana (it should be completely black or close to it)
- 1/2 cup coconut sugar
- 1 tsp vanilla extract
- 3/4 tsp coffee extract (optional)
- 1/2 tsp baking soda
- 1/2 tsp fine sea salt
- 1/2 tsp ground cinnamon
- 3/4 cup oat flour
- 3/4 cup rolled oats
- 3/4 cup almond flour
- 1 tbsp arrowroot powder
- 1/3 cup sundried bananas, cubed
- 1/4 cup + 1 tbsp dark chocolate chips, divided

Instructions

1. In a large mixing bowl, mash the banana with a fork.
2. Add coconut sugar and beat with a hand mixer until combined.
3. Add in the flax egg, vanilla extract and coffee extract and beat until combined.
4. Add the baking soda, salt and cinnamon and beat again.
5. In a medium bowl, mix oat flour, rolled oats, almond flour and arrowroot powder. Add to the wet ingredient and beat until combined.
6. Stir in sundried banana and the 1/4 cup of chocolate chips.
7. Spoon dough into prepared pan and spread out until smooth and mostly even. Since the dough is sticky, covering the dough with a piece of parchment paper helps to spread it (I cover with parchment paper and spread with my hands).
8. Sprinkle the remaining 1 tbsp of chocolate chips on top and press down.
9. Bake for 18-20 minutes, until lightly golden and firm to the touch.
10. Place pan on a cooling rack for 10 minutes.

11. Lift square out and place directly on the cooling rack
for 20 minutes, until cool.

12. Slice in four in each direction to have 12 squares.

29. Cauliflower Vegan Bolognese

Prep Time: 10 Minutes

Cook Time: 60 Minutes

Serving: 5

Ingredients

- 1 tbsp virgin coconut oil
- 3 cloves garlic, pressed
- 1 carrot, chopped
- 5 cups chopped cauliflower
- 1/2 cup packed spinach, coarsely chopped
- 1 tomato, seeded and chopped
- 1/4 cup sundried tomatoes, finely chopped
- 1 tbsp capers
- 1 can (14 oz) no-salt-added crushed tomatoes
- 2 cups tomato soup or tomato sauce
- 2 tbsp tomato paste
- 2 tsp dried basil
- 1 tsp dried oregano
- salt and pepper to taste

Instructions

1. Heat oil in a large pot over medium heat. Add garlic, carrot, cauliflower and spinach and cook, stirring, until the spinach is wilted. Add all remaining ingredients, stir and bring to a boil. Reduce heat to low, cover, and let cook 1 hour. Remove from heat and either blend a little with a hand held mixer or transfer to a blender and pulse a couple times until you reach desired consistency.
2. Serve with zucchini noodles, spaghetti squash or your choice of whole grain pasta.

30. Carrot & Broccoli Mac N' Cheese

Prep Time: 5 Minutes

Cook Time: 60 Minutes

Serving: 6

Ingredients

- 7 carrots, peeled and coarsely chopped
- 1 broccoli, in small florets
- 1 tbsp olive oil
- 1 white onion, chopped
- 1 package (375 g) whole wheat elbow macaroni
- 2 slices of bread (I used sprouted bread)
- 2 tbsp softened butter or non-hydrogenated margarine, divided
- 1 tbsp flour
- 1 1/4 cup warm milk (I used 1%)
- 1/2 package Maclaren's Imperial Sharp Cold Pack Cheddar
- 1/4 cup grated parmesan
- 1/2 tsp dry yellow mustard
- 1 tsp salted herbs, or salt to taste
- Paprika

Instructions

1. Bring a pot of water to a boil. Add carrots and cook until tender. Remove carrots with a slotted spoon and place in a bowl. Add broccoli to the water and cook for 1-2 minutes until crisp-tender. Mash or puree the carrots (it is fine if there's a few chunks) and set aside.

2. Heat olive oil in a skillet over medium heat. Cook onion until translucent. Remove from heat and set aside.

3. Bring a big pot of water to a boil and cook macaroni according to package directions.

4. Meanwhile, process the two slices of bread in a food processor until coarse crumbs start to form. Add 1 tbsp softened butter and process until combined. Set aside.

5. In a large saucepan, melt remaining 1 tbsp of butter over medium heat. Add flour and stir with a whisk until it starts to bubble. Gradually whisk in milk, then stir constantly until the sauce starts to thicken, about 5 minutes. Add both cheeses and stir until completely melted. Stir in mashed carrots, dry mustard and salted herbs. Toss the drained macaroni, the broccoli florets and the cooked onions in the sauce.

www.ingramcontent.com/pod-product-compliance
Lightning Source LLC
Chambersburg PA
CBHW050053260726
48658CB00005B/1933